CBD & Cannabis Oil
The Essential Guide

by Oscar Bailey

Table of Contents

Additionally, the information in the following pages is intended only for informational purposes and should thus be thought of as universal. As befitting its nature, it is presented without assurance regarding its prolonged validity or interim quality. Trademarks that are mentioned are done without written consent and can in no way be considered an endorsement from the trademark holder.

Introduction: Cannabis Basics

*Congratulations on downloading **CBD & Cannabis Oil: The Essential Guide**. We are confident that this book will teach you everything you need to know about cannabis oil, CBD and cannabis products, and that it will answer any questions that you may have—especially in regards to the legalities surrounding Cannabis products. There are many books available on this subject, and we are so happy you have chosen ours! If you find this book helpful or informative, please consider leaving us an honest review on Amazon.*

Marijuana is a controversial topic. In the United States, it is now legal in many states for medical use, and legal in a few states for recreational use, but it is not legal in *all* states. If you are reading this book, you probably do not know much about marijuana or its derivatives, their history, their legal status, or the wide variety of uses they have—especially in medicine. Before we begin, we should point out that marijuana, cannabis, and hemp all refer to the same product. Traditionally, marijuana has been known as a psychoactive drug meant to "get you high." Cannabis usually refers to the plant that marijuana comes from, and hemp refers to the parts of that plant that are *not* psychoactive or high-inducing. There are many different names for the plant and all of its forms, and we realize it can be difficult to differentiate one name from another. The most important thing you should know going forward is that THC is the compound that "gets you high," and CBD is a similar compound that does *not* induce psychoactive or psychotropic results. But we will explain that later!

First, let us start by discussing what is legal and where.

There are two types of marijuana use recognized by state governments here in the U.S. — "Medical Marijuana" and "Recreational Marijuana." Some states allow both, some states only allow Medical use and some states prohibit all marijuana use.

Medical Marijuana is legal in the following states:

- *Washington D.C.*
- *Washington*
- *Vermont*
- *Rhode Island*
- *Pennsylvania*
- *Oregon*
- *Ohio*
- *North Dakota*
- *New York*
- *New Mexico*
- *New Jersey*
- *New Hampshire*
- *Nevada*
- *Montana*
- *Minnesota*
- *Michigan*
- *Massachusetts*
- *Maryland*
- *Maine*
- *Illinois*
- *Hawaii*
- *Florida*
- *Delaware*
- *Connecticut*
- *Colorado*
- *California*
- *Arkansas*
- *Arizona*
- *Alaska*
- In *West Virginia*, only cannabis-infused products are legal for medical use.
- In *Louisiana*, medical marijuana is legal in every form except those forms that can be smoked.

Recreational Marijuana is legal in the following states:

- *Washington D.C.*
- *Vermont*
- *Oregon*
- *Nevada*
- *Massachusetts*
- *Maine*
- *Colorado*
- *California*
- *Alaska*

Marijuana— whether medical or recreational—is illegal in the following states:

- *Wyoming*
- *Wisconsin*
- *Virginia*
- *Utah*
- *Texas*
- *Tennessee*
- *South Dakota*
- *South Carolina*
- *Oklahoma*
- *North Carolina*
- *Nebraska*
- *Missouri*
- *Mississippi*
- *Kentucky*
- *Kansas*
- *Iowa*
- *Indiana*
- *Idaho*
- *Georgia*
- *Alabama*

- In *Alabama* and *Mississippi*, medical marijuana can be prescribed and used in cases of severe epilepsy, but it is nearly impossible to obtain that diagnosis.

On a Federal level, all marijuana use is still illegal. For the most part, federal prosecution of marijuana-use is not a concern in states that have legalized it. But if you legally purchase Marijuana in Nevada, and then cross state lines with it into Utah, you could be facing a wealth of legal trouble, including charges of possession, trafficking, and more. Federal law also prohibits federal employees from using marijuana even if they live in a state that has legalized it.

Now, it is important to note that not all marijuana products are illegal. Marijuana can be broken down to its chemical properties, and many of those properties are completely legal to use in every state and on a federal level.

The two main compounds in marijuana are the cannabinoids THC and CBD. THC leads to intoxication, while CBD does not. Many studies have shown that CBD extracts have anti-inflammatory properties, and can be useful in treating both anxiety and seizure disorders.

As more and more states have legalized marijuana use, many new CBD products have arrived on the market—from oils to tinctures, to lozenges, to dog treats. Each state handles CBD products differently. Some classify it the same way they classify marijuana and therefore require a valid Medical Marijuana card to purchase CBD products. Other states do not classify CBD extract as a drug, and can, therefore, sell CBD products over the counter to anyone.

The federal government classifies CBD exactly as they classify Marijuana. Therefore, CBD products cannot be purchased online and shipped across state lines. If you find a CBD product online, do your research and ask questions. If the product is not manufactured and distributed within the same state as you, then it probably is not a true CBD product, and it may be mislabeled.

The Attorney General of the United States, Jeff Sessions, has made many statements—as has the Drug Enforcement Agency (or DEA)—about CBD Oil and cannabis, and much of what they have had to say was false. Their statements are designed as "scare tactics," to prevent people from pursuing CBD Oil use.

Remember, whether the product is called cannabis, hemp, marijuana, or any of the other colloquial terms, it all comes from the exact same plant: *Cannabis sativa* or *Cannabis indica*. Some of the "street names" for marijuana/cannabis include:

- Weed
- Thai Stick
- Texas Tea
- Stinkweed
- Skunk
- Rope
- Reefer
- Pot
- Panama Gold
- Nuggets
- Mexican
- Maui Wowie
- Mary Jane
- Joint
- Indo
- Herb
- Hay
- Green Tobacco
- Grass
- Gangster
- Ganga
- Dope
- Colombo
- Chronic
- Charge
- Cannabis
- Burrito
- Burnie
- Buds
- Broccoli
- Boom
- Boo
- Blunt
- Block
- Blaze
- Black Russian
- Ashes
- Acapulco Gold
- 420

Are hemp and cannabis different? They are! Hemp refers to a cannabis product that contains less than 0.3% of the THC cannabinoid. Hemp products are *legal* under federal law for both academic and educational purposes. If a product is referred to as Cannabis, it must contain more than 0.3% of the THC cannabinoid.

The Agricultural Act of 2014, signed into law by President Obama, included a section that specifically defined the difference between marijuana and "industrial hemp." This definition can be found in Section 7606 of the act, titled *Legitimacy of Industrial Hemp Research*. This act—and definition—authorized the research on industrial hemp to be performed by "institutions of higher education" (i.e., universities), as well as by the agricultural departments of state governments. This allows each state to regulate industrial and industrial hemp research, without interference from the federal government.

Without this piece of legislation, CBD Oil would be even more controversial than it already is. As it stands, this legislation dictates that because the plant itself is legal (when the THC level is less than 0.3%), then any product made from that plant is also legal (as long as it has less than 0.3% THC).

In the United States, there are thirty-three states that have hemp-specific legislation. These states are:

- West Virginia
- Washington
- Virginia
- Vermont
- Utah
- Tennessee
- South Carolina
- Rhode Island
- Pennsylvania
- Oregon
- North Dakota
- North Carolina
- New York
- New Hampshire
- Nevada
- Nebraska
- Montana
- Missouri
- Minnesota
- Michigan
- Maryland
- Maine
- Kentucky
- Indiana
- Illinois
- Hawaii
- Florida
- Delaware
- Connecticut
- Colorado
- California
- Alabama

Of those thirty-three states, only fourteen of them allow the production of hemp seeds for use in academic and industrial settings. These fourteen states are:

- West Virginia
- Virginia
- Vermont
- Tennessee
- South Carolina
- Oregon
- North Dakota
- North Carolina
- Missouri
- Massachusetts
- Kentucky
- Indiana
- Colorado
- California

Because these states have only been producing hemp seeds for a few years, the standard preference is still to use European-sourced hemp seeds for research and industrial use.

Meanwhile, in 2017, the federal government passed an Appropriations bill that specifically prevents the Department of Justice from establishing new laws or legislation that may authorize the "use, distribution, possession or cultivated of medical marijuana." While hemp is *not* medical marijuana, it is still legal (along with the extracted non-THC), but the federal government is currently prohibited from authorizing the use of medical marijuana.

Hemp or CBD products have actually been on the market for a number of years, and while we are only now discovering just how useful these products may be for our daily lives, they have actually been used in various cultures for many, many centuries. Not only can you purchase CBD-infused lotions, shampoos, clothes, shoes and more, but it can also even be used to help reduce the level of radiation emitted from nuclear waste.

Did you know that hemp crops or cannabis crops use half the water than standard crops like wheat, and these crops can be grown without the use of pesticides? This is incredibly important, especially for those that are concerned with the health of the environment. It is a more sustainable crop, and it is safer to grow, use, and consume. What's more is that hemp or cannabis is a good source of fiber, and the seeds are rich in proteins and omegas, as well vitamins, antioxidants, and other nutrients.

When marketed as a dietary supplement, hemp is completely legal throughout the United States. Many of these "dietary supplements" are also used as nutritional supplements or vitamins. This is accomplished by pairing CBD with other vitamins, fatty acids, minerals, terpenes, other trace cannabinoids, and flavonoids. When categorized as a "dietary supplement," the product must comply with the Food & Drug Administration's guidelines, and the manufacturer is then prohibited from endorsing or promoting the CBD-specific benefits of the product. In addition, these "dietary supplements" cannot recommend a particular daily intake. It is up to the consumer to determine if the product is right for them.

In most cases, CBD and other cannabinoids are legal in the United States—as long as they do not contain THC. Transporting these products across state lines, or shipping them over state lines, can complicate the legalities of the issue. Continue reading for more information on CBD and the many medical benefits and uses of this incredible cannabinoid.

What do you know about the history of hemp? Let us discuss it!

Over 10,000 years ago, weaving hemp fiber was recorded for the first time. Carbon testing of archaeological artifacts has found wild hemp strains that date a far back as 8000 B.C. The cultivation of hemp dates back as far as 800 A.D. in Great Britain. It was heavily encouraged by King Henry VIII in the 16th century that farmers plant hemp crops to provide extensive material for the British Naval fleet. The British Naval fleet needed the hemp supply to construct the battleships, riggings, pennants, pendants, oakum, and sails. They even used hemp paper for logs, maps, and bibles. Hemp was a vital part of the sailors' everyday lives.

In colonial America, during the 17th century, farmers in Connecticut, Massachusetts, and Virginia were actually ordered by law to begin growing an Indian strain of hemp. Colonial laws dictated that if a member of the colony was not using part of their land to grow hemp, they could actually be fined and sentenced to jail. Hemp was even used in bartering situation as a legal tender. It was even acceptable as a tax payment. By 1850, nearly 8500 hemp plantations of 2000 acres or more were listed on the United States census. They were planting everything from China hemp to Japanese hemp to Smyrna hemp.

Harvesting was typically done with a hand brake operated machine until a machine was finally built that processed the hemp entirely—from breaking the retted stalks to cleaning the fiber, and finally, to producing consistent hemp fiber. This machine could process and harvest more than a thousand pounds of clean, usable hemp fiber every hour. Thanks to this machine, hemp cultivation was finally a financially attractive option for farmers and went far in reducing labor costs. By 1920, nearly all hemp crops were harvested with this machine.

In addition to hemp fiber, hemp was also used as a fuel source. Henry Ford, the founder of Ford Motor Company, established and operated a biomass fuel conversion plant that used hemp to produce hemp oil. He did this to compete with Rudolph Diesel, who engineered the famous diesel engine in 1896, with the intention of using a variety of biofuels to fuel the engine. Industries that were competing with hemp fuel panicked at this latest innovation and began a smear campaign that insisted hemp was the same product as marijuana. A propaganda film called *Reefer Madness* was produced to stop hemp production.

The public quickly began to associate hemp with the intoxicating properties of THC, and in 1937, the Marijuana Tax Act was passed by the United States Congress. This act was a major factor in the decline of hemp production, as new regulations requiring licensing and additional taxing of hemp cultivation made it nearly impossible for farmers in America to harvest hemp.

Despite the new belief that hemp was a "taboo" or an inappropriate product, it became incredibly important during World War II. Because of the attack on Pearl Harbor by the Japanese, the United States was unable to import Manila hemp from the Philippine islands. Without this imported hemp, the United States Drug Administration began to reconsider their stance on hemp. They produced and released their own "propaganda" film called *Hemp for Victory*, which was meant to encourage the production of hemp among American farmers. They branded hemp production as a "war effort," and they even created a private government program called War Hemp Industries, which worked to subsidize the growth and cultivation of hemp. One million acres of land in the Midwest was purchased by the program and used specifically for the growth and cultivation of hemp. Unfortunately, a soon as World War II ended, all of the hemp farms and hemp processing plants were shut down, and the new industry disappeared just as quickly as it was brought back to life. Today, wild hemp can be found scattered all over the Midwest United States.

As a result of the "war effort" hemp production, the United States government began to recognize "industrial hemp" as a product differentiated from marijuana. This went on from 1937 until the late 1960s, when the Controlled Substances Act was passed by the United States Congress. When that act was passed, hemp became an illegal product yet again, as it was no longer recognized for its distinctions from marijuana.

Obviously, we have made greater strides when it comes to legalizing marijuana and hemp (or cannabis), but there is still a long, legal road ahead. Someday, we are sure, marijuana will be legal for both medical and recreational use, and there will be no question *anywhere* about the legality of hemp or cannabis products.

Glossary of Important Terms

Cannabinoid: compounds of the cannabis plant that can be extracted for medicinal use.

Cannabis: a tall, stiff plant with serrated leaves; the plant itself can be broken down and used for hemp products, while the flower and leaves can be dried and are more colloquially known as marijuana.

CBC: one of the four primary cannabinoid compounds, considered non-intoxicating.

CBD: one of the four primary cannabinoid compounds, considered non-intoxicating.

CBG: one of the four primary cannabinoid compounds, considered non-intoxicating.

Endocannabinoid System: a naturally-occurring part of the body's immune system which responds to cannabinoids and produces cannabinoids on its own.

Hemp: this is the fibrous part of the plant that is used for hemp products and the part of the plant that CBD is typically extracted from. Hemp is non-intoxicating.

THC: one of the four primary cannabinoid compounds, considered to be intoxicating when concentrated in amounts higher than 0.3%.

Marijuana: the flowering part of the cannabis plant that has intoxicating or "psychoactive" properties.

Chapter 1: Varieties of Cannabis

Cannabinoids is the term used to describe the different compounds found in marijuana or cannabis. There are four major cannabinoids, and each one has slightly different properties.

- THC
- CBD
- CBG
- CBC

As we mentioned before, **THC** is the compound responsible for "getting you high." THC was first isolated from the cannabis plant in 1964 by an Israeli chemist named Raphael Mechoulam. His research led to the discovery of other cannabinoids and the many potential uses for cannabis products.

Cannabinoids actually have no role in the development of the plant. They are secondary metabolites and simply act as the plant's immune system. Scientists suspect that this is why cannabinoids have so many healthy properties.

THC, in particular, binds to the cannabinoid receptors in the brain and works with your central nervous system to produce "psychoactive effects." Everyone responds to THC in a different manner—some experience calm and peaceful feelings, while others may experience an increase in paranoia or anxiety. This can depend not only on your own body chemistry but also on which strain or what concentration of THC you have consumed.

If you have a negative experience with one particular strain, or with a high concentration, it may be worth trying a different strain or a lower concentration. The recommendation is always to start on the low end and to take it slow. It is important to remember that a cannabis high will not only last for several hours, but it may also take several hours to take effect. If you do not feel anything after thirty minutes, give yourself more time. Do not immediately consume more, assuming that it is not working. It is, it may just need more time.

Various strains and concentrations of THC are known for inducing the following short-term effects:

- sedation
- relaxation
- red eyes
- paranoia
- pain relief
- memory impairment
- laughter
- increased heart rate
- hunger
- feeling heavy
- energy
- elation
- dry mouth
- drowsiness
- dizziness
- anxiety

Long-term effects of THC are not well-documented or well-researched. It is suspected that THC may cause anatomical changes to the brain, bronchitis, poor memory, and/or psychosis. Chronic THC use may also lead to an increased tolerance for THC, which may lead to increased use.

One recent study suggested that THC can alter the Corpus Callosum, which is the part of the brain that connects the right and left side (or cerebral hemispheres). Participants in the study that reported daily use of high concentrations of THC had measurable changes in the Corpus Callosum, but the study could not identify what those changes meant.

Bronchitis is listed as a long-term side effect if the THC is consumed via inhalation of the smoke. This side effect is part of the reason THC-infused products have become incredibly popular—including THC vapor.

Memory can also be affected by chronic THC use. In March 2016, one study was released that suggested THC use could lead to decreased cognitive function, especially in terms of verbal skills. The study suggested that for every five years of chronic cannabis or THC use, participants would forget one word from a list of fifteen. However, this study was not independently verified, and the sample size of participants was very small.

Some studies have also suggested that chronic THC use may lead to psychosis, but only in participants that were already predisposed to psychotic disorders like schizophrenia. Studies have suggested that those who are predisposed to these disorders may develop symptoms three to five years earlier than they would have if they had *not* consumed cannabis or THC.

And of course, chronic use of any substance, intoxicating or otherwise, can lead to a higher tolerance of that substance. Having a higher tolerance inevitably means it will take more and more of that substance to achieve the desired effect.

Many THC studies have also ruled out both overdose and cancer as side effects. No evidence has been shown to support implications that THC use can increase your risk of cancer, and there has never been a documented case of THC overdose or THC-related fatality.

The suspected medicinal benefits of THC far outweigh the risks or "side effects." THC is thought to have a positive effect on the following conditions:

- Sleep Apnea
- PTSD
- Neuropathic Pain
- Nausea
- Fibromyalgia
- Crohn's Disease
- Chronic Pain
- Cancer
- Arthritis

- Multiple Sclerosis (MS)
- Migraines
- Insomnia
- Inflammation
- Glaucoma

- Appetite Loss
- Alzheimer's
- ADHD

As we mentioned before, there has been little research into THC and cannabis use as it was prohibited for so many years. Now that the legality of the product is changing, research on the product will become more popular, and we are likely to learn quite a bit about the medical benefits, side effects and more.

The most common way to ingest THC is by smoking marijuana or cannabis. When cannabis is heated, decarboxylation occurs. Without the decarboxylation, cannabis is actually non-intoxicating. THC can be heated by cooking it or lighting it in a pipe or other smoking mechanism. Not everyone enjoys smoking THC, especially if they are not accustomed to smoking cigarettes, cigars or other substances. Smoking THC can be very harsh and can produce an uncomfortable cough. For those that do not want to smoke THC, it may be wise to invest in edible THC products. With edibles, the decarboxylation occurred when the edible was cooked or baked. Therefore, it is just as intoxicating as the smoked variety. In some cases, many people even find edible THC to be *more* intoxicating than smoked THC.

Now, you may want to know what the difference is between the THC and CBD. We discussed earlier that THC is the property that produces the "high." CBD does not have the same psychoactive effect as THC.

CBD is thought to have same effects on inflammation, pain, and anxiety, in addition to other medical benefits, but none of the intoxicating effects. This is why CBD can be sold over-the-counter or without a Medical Marijuana card in some states.

It is important to remember that CBD is completely inert, this means you will not experience the sensations or feelings of "being stoned." Because CBD is not intoxicating, products that contain CBD only (products without any THC), are not subjected to the same regulations as those that contain THC. CBD products are often referred to as "hemp products," rather than "cannabis products" or "marijuana products."

Even in the states that do *not* allow medical or recreational marijuana use, some laws allow the purchase and use of CBD-only products. These products may not be easy to find or obtain, but they are legal if they are truly free of THC.

If either medical or recreational marijuana is legal in your state, then it is a guarantee that CBD products are not only legal but easily accessible. While they may not be sold at your local pharmacy, they should be available over-the-counter at any marijuana dispensary, and they should be available for purchase without a Medical Marijuana card.

CBD can be extracted from both hemp plants and marijuana plants. When it is extracted from a marijuana plant, it typically contains a trace amount of THC. The level of THC will determine whether that particular extraction is legal or not, and whether or not it is subject to the same regulations as true THC products.

Most states require the THC level to be less than 1%, while other states require less than 0.3%. Delaware currently allows up to 5% THC in CBD products, and while 5% still is not even enough to cause intoxication, that is currently the highest legal limit for CBD products.

Studies have shown that CBD sourced from marijuana plants is more potent than CBD sourced from hemp, but both are effective. CBD is considered most effective when it is derived from marijuana simply because there are other "companion cannabinoids" that it can work with and that will make it more effective. The companion cannabinoids do not exist in hemp plants, but there are a plethora of them in marijuana plants.

The strongest and most commonly recommended CBD strains available are Harlequin, Katelyn Faith, Remedy, ACDC, Cannatonic, and Charlotte's Web. These strains contain high levels of CBD, but they also contain high levels of THC, which makes them legal for those with Medical Marijuana cards and those that live in a state with Recreational Marijuana. In terms of their medicinal benefits, they are the best. But they may not be available to you over-the-counter.

In terms of the medicinal benefits of CBD, let us first discuss how CBD works in our bodies, and why it works.

First, each person has a network of neurons within their body that is referred to as the "endocannabinoid system." This system contains a wealth of receptions that bind to the cannabinoids you ingest, like CBD. Not much is known about the connections and interactions between these receptors, and so many of the physical responses we may experience are actually unknown and/or undocumented.

The endocannabinoid system within your body is connected to every other major system of our body. This why marijuana and cannabis have such a wide-ranging list of medicinal benefits and effects. Every part of your body responds to marijuana or cannabis and likewise responds to CBD.

Research into the effect and benefits of cannabis is still limited, but now that the legalities surrounding the issue are changing and perhaps relaxing, there is sure to be a wealth of new research with each passing year. We will undoubtedly discover that marijuana or cannabis use can affect even more than we already know.

One study has shown that CBD may be an incredibly effective treatment for epilepsy and similar seizure disorders. In 2012, the British Epilepsy Association published a study that strongly supported CBD as a therapeutic mechanism for epilepsy of all kinds. The name of this study is "Cannabidiol exert anticonvulsant effects in animal models temporal lobe and partial seizures." This study is widely available online, and we strongly recommend that you read it if you are at all skeptical about CBD and the effect it may have on seizure disorders.

In addition, researchers have found that CBD may be beneficial in the treatment of neurological diseases, from Parkinson's to Multiple Sclerosis to Alzheimer's. These conditions are not well understood, and there are few (if any) treatments for them, but a 2006 study suggested that Alzheimer's, in particular, is directly linked to a protein pathway in our brain.

Scientists have found that, on a molecular level, CBD may have a protective effect on nerve cells, and may prevent or slow down degenerative disorders. This is called the "neuroprotective effect." Because CBD can have this effect, it makes perfect sense that CBD may be a great tool in the fight neurodegenerative disorders.

Most commonly, though, CBD is used to treat pain. It has become a popular alternative or opioids and other prescription painkillers, especially as the opioid-epidemic continues to increase, and restrictions on opioid prescription continue to increase, as well.

A study from 2015 compared the pain-relieving properties of CBD to that of morphine, and it was even found to work well in conjunction with morphine, allowing smaller doses of morphine to be prescribed. It also assisted in reducing the side effects of morphine.

Better yet, a 2015 study found that CBD oil can inhibit tumor growth. Patients in the study experienced slower cancer growth, whether they had lung cancer, prostate cancer, breast cancer, colon cancer, or other types of cancer.

You see, CBD makes it difficult for cancer cells to grow, and in many cases, this actually leads to the death of cancer cells, as they rely on rapid regeneration. If they cannot regenerate, they cannot overwhelm the immune system. If they cannot overwhelm the immune system, the immune system is far more likely to fight them off and win the battle.

Furthermore, CBD and THC each have anti-inflammatory properties, and CBD has more of these properties than THC. Your endocannabinoid system binds with CBD and creates an anti-inflammatory response directed specifically at your nerves. This is yet another neuroprotective quality, and it is the main reason that CBD is now being used to treat neurological disorders.

Now, can CBD also be used to treat emotional issues or mood disorders?

In the United States, nearly eight percent of the population is affected by Post-Traumatic Stress Disorder (or PTSD), and that number climbs every year. Men are less likely to suffer from PTSD than women, but regardless of gender, it can be incredibly difficult and expensive to find an effective treatment for Post-Traumatic Stress Disorder.

In 2013, one study found that the use of CBD may improve a person's ability to forget a traumatic memory or event. While this study did not conclude that the CBD permanently erased these traumatic memories, it did suggest that it made it easier for those suffering from Post-Traumatic Stress Disorder to "let go of" or stop focusing on traumatic memories. This study was groundbreaking and may provide the necessary foundation for future CBD or cannabis studies.

CBD is also commonly used to treat other emotional issues or mood disorders like anxiety, depression, agoraphobia, and more. Just as CBD can calm physical inflammation, they also have a calming effect on the mind and can assist in the product of serotonin and other "happy" brain chemicals.

Now that we have discussed the medicinal, emotional and physical benefits of CBD, we should discuss whether or not CBD is used recreationally, and why.

As we previously discussed, CBD is not intoxicating like THC. Because of this, CBD is the perfect counterweight to intoxicating THC. Using the two together can ensure that you do not get experience too much of a high or too much intoxication.

Some people have reported anxiety or paranoia when they use THC. This negative experience may be helped by increasing the amount of CBD that is ingested along with the THC. Some people may describe this as an "easier trip." The overall experience is meant to be softer and more pleasant, which is important for those people that might be more sensitive to the effects of THC. Remember, everyone responds to THC differently.

If you are lucky enough to live in a state that allows recreational marijuana, go to a local dispensary and look closely at the products they sell. You will notice that nearly all of the THC products also include high quantities of CBD.

Speaking of CBD products, there are several different varieties in which CBD can be purchased. First—and by far the most popular—is CBD oil. These oils can be infused into both health and beauty products, from topical ointments that are absorbed through the skin, to moisturizers, shampoos, deodorant, and even facial cleansers.

CBD Oil can also be used with a vaporizer. It is usually compressed into a wax form, which is then placed in a small cartridge that is warmed by a battery. As the wax melts, it creates a vapor that can then be inhaled. This is much like the nicotine vaporizers available on the market today.

Finally, CBD oil can be used in edible products, from foods to beverages to tinctures. Tinctures refer to a flavored oil, which is typically applied to your tongue or under your tongue by drops.

Edible products are extremely popular, from cookies and candy bars to lozenges to drinks. Edible products are easy to consume, and the cannabis or cannabinoids in them are nearly impossible to taste.

In addition, CBD oils are now being used in pet products. CBD dog treats are popular and can be used to treat anything from joint pain to anxiety and more. CBD powders, usually flavored, are also popular, as they can be sprinkled on the food of a particularly picky dog.

There are a wealth of CBD products available, but it is important to remember that you need to do your research. Some companies will imply the presence of CBD or THC when none truly exists. In addition, CBD products will rarely be available for purchase online. You will almost always need to purchase CBD products from a medical or recreational dispensary.

As you have now learned, the potential for CBD is endless, and we are surely only at the beginning of the science or research behind it. We will discover so much more about CBD and the medicinal properties of it over the next decade, and CBD use is sure to become more mainstream. From slowing the progression of cancer to reducing anxiety and depression, to relieving pain and inflammation, it is pretty safe to say that CBD is a "miracle drug." And to think it is even all-natural!

Finally, we should discuss the **CBC** and **CBG** cannabinoid properties of marijuana or cannabis, beginning with CBC.

CBC is a cannabinoid known as cannabichromene. Little is known about CBC, but research shows that it has a promising future. Fifty years ago, CBC was discovered as one of the cannabinoids that branch off from the CBG that is produced by cannabis plants. Like CBD, CBC is non-intoxicating. It does not bind well to the CB1 cannabinoid receptor in our endocannabinoid system. Therefore, a euphoric high is experienced when CBC is ingested. However, it does bind well to two pain receptors, the transient receptor potential ankyrin (or TRPA1) and the vanilloid receptor (or TRPV1). These receptors are linked to our mind's perception of pain. When these receptors bind to CBC, our bodies automatically release all-natural endocannabinoids like anandamide.

Researchers in the midst of studying CBC all agree—CBC works best when it is paired with other cannabinoids, like CBD and THC. While it does work independently, it is most effective when it is working with a team of other cannabinoids to produce the desired effect.

As we know from our discussion of CBD, researchers are now finding that cannabinoids are effective in the fight against cancer. While they have yet to be found curative, they do seem to have a substantial effect on the speed in which cancer spreads. CBC or CBD use will slow the progression of cancer, and it will allow anandamide to work longer and harder within our bloodstream. Anandamide is known as the "bliss molecule," and is actually your body's natural version of THC.

One recent study actually documented a significant decrease in the growth of a tumor on a mouse with skin carcinogenesis. The cannabinoids not only slowed down the rate of tumor growth, but it also inhibited the inflammation present.

Another study has shown that Anandamide, independent of cannabinoid use, has been a key component in the fight against breast cancer. Logically, if Anandamide can assist in the fight against cancer, and CBC helps Anandamide work longer and harder, then CBC may be one of the best cancer treatments available.

A study published in 2006 found that CBC is actually an incredibly potent cannabinoid when it comes to preventing or slowing down the growth and development of new cancer cells. CBG, which we will discuss next, was found to be the single most effective cannabinoid, with CBC placing a close second.

In addition, CBC has been shown to relieve osteoarthritis inflammation and pain—and without the same side effects of non-steroidal anti-inflammatories (or NSAIDs).

CBC cannabinoids can even assist in healthy brain function! A study from 2013 found that CBC improved the performance of neural stem progenitor cells (or NSPCs). These cells differentiate into something called an astroglial cell. Astroglial cells are vital in maintaining brain homeostasis, as they are responsible for neurotransmitter direction, defending your brain and body against oxidative stress, reducing inflammation, and assisting in detoxification.

Some studies have also shown that CBC can help fight acne. Acne occurs when your skin produces an overabundance of sebum, leading to inflamed sebaceous glands. CBC, with their anti-inflammatory properties, can suppress the inflammation of the sebaceous glands, as well as suppress the production of excessive lipids. Furthermore, CBC also reduces the levels of arachidonic acid. Arachidonic acid is necessary for creating lipogenesis, which is a major contributing factor in the presence of acne.

As we discussed before, both CBD and THC can have a powerful effect on depression. Studies are now showing that CBC also has powerful effects on depression, especially when used in conjunction with CBD, THC or both. Not much research on CBC has been done, but the research already done has been promising.

Finally, let us discuss the fourth and final of the major cannabinoids. CBG is found in much smaller quantities than other cannabinoids in marijuana and cannabis. Like CBD and CBC, CBG is non-intoxicating. In most strains of cannabis, there is only one percent or less of the CBG cannabinoid present. But with cannabis products becoming more and more popular, we are sure to see new hybrids and strains reach the market that container higher and higher levels of CBG.

CBG responds to heat like the other cannabinoids do, but they respond best to ultraviolet light. As new strains are being developed, cannabis breeders are using genetic manipulation and plant cross-breeding to achieve higher yields of CBG in these new strains.

Scientists are also finding success in extracting higher and higher levels of CBG by extracting them from the budding plant instead of the flowering plant. They do this by pinpointing the "optimum extraction time," which is typically within seven to nine weeks into the flowering cycle of the plant. For example, the medicinal strain known as Bediol is being bred by a company called Bedrocan BV Medicinal Cannabis.

CBG works in just the same way that the other cannabinoids work, they interact with the endocannabinoid system that every human body is naturally equipped with. CBG is especially effective in the treatment of glaucoma and intraocular pressure. It also acts as a vasodilator and has many neuroprotective qualities.

Some animal studies have found that CBG can be effective in decreasing the inflammation associated with inflammatory bowel disease. A study from 2015 also found that CBG played a vital role in the treatment of mice with Huntington's disease, as the CBG prevented nerve cell degeneration within the brain and therefore acted as a neuroprotectant.

And, just as we have found with other cannabinoids (THC, CBD, and CBC), the CBG cannabinoid can be effective in the fight against cancer. Studies have shown that it can block the receptors that cause cancer cell growth and the progression of cancer. It has shown particular promise in slowing or inhibiting the growth of the cells involved in colorectal cancer. The CBG cannabinoid not only slowed down the growth of the tumors, but it also slowed down the growth of the colon carcinogenesis induced by chemicals. This information—and new cancer studies—mean that we soon see a true cure for colorectal cancer.

In addition, there has been a wealth of research in Europe that suggests the CBG cannabinoid has antibacterial properties, and that many of those antibacterial agents may be effective against the microbial strains of methicillin-resistant Staphylococcus aureus (or MRSA). In fact, topical ointments derived from or infused with cannabis have been used in Europe to treat various skin infections.

More recently, a 2017 study has shown that CBG can actually be used as an appetite stimulant. The hope is that extracting high concentrations of CBG may be useful in treating cachexia and the associated effects like the severe weight loss and muscle wasting that often occurs as cancer and other diseases progress. Also, CBG has also been shown to be effective in treating bladder dysfunction disorders by inhibiting muscle contractions.

The future of CBG cannabinoid research and the products may result from this research is promising. We are sure to learn so much more about CBG over the next few years, and scientists suspect that we will discover CBG to be helpful in treating psoriasis and other skin conditions, as an antidepressant, and even as an analgesic.

Ultimately, the possibilities are endless, and we are learning more and more every day about cannabinoids and the wide variety of medicinal benefits for these products. From THC to CBD to CBC to CBG, we are sure to discover that the various extracts of cannabis can be used to treat everything from cancer to anxiety to depression to everyday concern like acne and psoriasis.

Chapter 2: The Effects of Cannabis

Now that you know about how cannabis and cannabinoids like CBD can be used medicinally, we should discuss what the side effects of cannabinoid ingestion are.

THC ingestion typically results in a euphoric high, usually characterized by feelings of relaxation and the overall reduction of stress. Sometimes, the THC high can also lead to "alterations in perception" or hallucinations. THC will also reduce pain and may ease social anxiety, making it easier to enjoy socializing. For some people, THC use also leads to an increase in creativity or introspection.

CBD ingestion can take the edge off the effects of THC—when it is used with THC. CBD can prevent hallucinations from being unpleasant or causing paranoia. When used alone, CBD (and the other cannabidiols, CBC and CBG) can be very therapeutic. It can relieve pain or ease anxiety.

It is important to remember that each strain of cannabis is different. Some strains have different or more intense effects than other strains. Each strain is derived from one of two types of the cannabis plant, sativa or indica. Sativa strains are meant to be "fun," and are often paired with social engagements or creative endeavors. Meanwhile, indica strains are meant to promote relaxation, which can be useful for those with anxiety or depression and can be used to treat insomnia, post-traumatic stress disorder, and more.

Some of the medical and recreational effects of CBD use include:
- slower progression of cancer or disease
- relief of nausea
- relief of anxiety

- reduced intraocular pressure
- pain relief
- increased sociability
- increased sensation
- increased libido
- increased introspection
- increased agreeableness
- greater creativity
- euphoria
- a sense of well-being
- altered perception
- a feeling of calm

Some of the less-positive side effects are:
- red or irritated eyes
- panic attacks
- lethargy or ataxia
- increased thirst
- increased heart rate
- increased appetite
- forgetfulness
- dry mouth
- dry eye
- dizziness
- depersonalization
- coughing
- bronchitis
- anxiety or paranoia

It is important to note that while the medicinal benefits are well-documented, researched and reported, the associated side effects are incredibly rare. Most reports of these side effects come from people who have ingested too much, too quickly, or from people that are unusually sensitive to cannabis. For most people, the side effects of cannabis will be limited to the classic side effects that are so often joked about on television and in the movies. You may experience "the munchies," or an increase in your appetite, and you may experience dry mouth or dry eyes. This is completely normal.

It is also important to note that cannabis is not lethal unless you are allergic to it, and even then, it typically does not lead to death. Simply put, cannabis is one of the safest medicinal products on the market, and overdosing on cannabis is essentially impossible.

In terms of addiction, it is exceedingly rare for people to become truly addicted to marijuana or cannabis. Some may develop a dependency, especially if they are using it to treat an issue like insomnia. These people may find it impossible to sleep without the use of cannabis, but this dependency is not nearly as unhealthy as a dependency on alcohol, or sleeping pills would be. Physically, cannabis has never been shown to have negative effects on your liver or kidney, and—short of developing chronic bronchitis as a result of smoking cannabis (which can be avoided simply by switching to tinctures or edible products)—cannabis use really has no long-term health concerns.

Overall, cannabis is completely safe to use, especially when you compare it to the other products on the market that may be used to treat the same condition you are trying to treat.

Interested in using CBD oil or other CBD products for your dog? Many dog owners are now purchasing CBD products to assist in the treatment of their dog's pain or arthritis, epilepsy, anxiety, cancer, and even as an appetite stimulant.

Canine CBD products can be easily found at your local dispensary, and as they should not contain any THC, they should be perfectly legal for you to purchase over-the-counter, even if you do not have a Medical Marijuana Card.

CBD has been found to reduce the frequency of seizures in dogs, relieve or reduce the inflammation surrounding canine joints, eliminate nausea, relieve depression, reduce anxiety (especially in cases of separation anxiety or storm anxiety), and reduce destructive behaviors. Also, just as CBD is thought to prevent or slow down the progression of cancer in humans, the same can be said for cancer in canine patients. It can slow it down or even possibly stop it. The effect CBD has on cancer is the same effect it has on other diseases, including autoimmune conditions, neurodegenerative conditions, inflammatory bowel disease, and cardiovascular (heart) disease.

CBD products have been available for dogs for a long time, and they are often marketed as "hemp products," as that is easier to market than "CBD products." Remember, hemp products or CBD products do not contain THC (or contain less than 0.3% THC), and as a result, these products are non-intoxicating.

So, can your dog use marijuana the way people do? Technically, yes. However, dogs process or metabolize marijuana differently than humans do, and it actually lasts in their system a whole lot longer than it lasts in a human's system. Even the smallest amount of marijuana or THC can last four or five times longer in your dog's body than in your own. Because of this, we *strongly* recommend that you purchase a CBD product specifically meant to be used in dogs. A human product may be too strong and may result in you having to hospitalize your pet at a veterinary facility, which may or may not feel obligated to report the incident to the authorities.

So, what kind of CBD product should you purchase for your dog? That genuinely depends on your dog's tastes and preferences. Canine CBD products are usually available as tinctures, powder-filled capsules, flavored powder (meant to be sprinkled on top of their food), topical ointments or creams, edible or flavored oils, or the classic dog treat. CBD oils and tinctures can be very bitter, no matter how they are flavored so a dog treat may be your safest bet, especially when you first start treating your pet with CBD products.

In addition, make sure that any CBD product you purchase for your pet does not contain an artificial sweetener called Xylitol. This sweetener is used in many CBD products for human consumption, and it is toxic to dogs. Even a tiny amount of Xylitol could lead to your dog's death. And, as always, you may want to discuss CBD products with your pet's veterinarian. In many cases, a prescription medication may be more appropriate, or it may need to be given in conjunction with a CBD product. Many communities now have "holistic" or "naturopathic" veterinarians as well, and they are the ones most likely to know which CBD products may be best for your pet, and where those products can be purchased.

If you are interested in trying a CBD product for your dog, we recommend using one of the products developed by Therabis, a company founded by a Veterinarian. Therabis provides several different product lines containing CBD: one line is tailored toward relieving anxiety, one is tailored toward relieving joint pain, and one is tailored toward reducing allergies. Each product line contains single-use or single-serve packets of the CBD product that can be sprinkled on your pet's food. Typically, your pet will only need one dose per day. They have also recently developed several types of pet treats within the same product lines.

TESTIMONIAL

Erin's dog, Toby, was rescued from a small humane society. Toby was young, physically healthy, and very sweet, but from the very beginning, Toby suffered from severe anxiety. He was afraid of new people, and Erin had to introduce him very slowly to new friends. He was afraid of new sounds and would panic any time a car backfired, or stormy weather arrived. He was even afraid to be alone and would become destructive if he was left home alone for more than an hour.

Erin tried everything. She crate-trained him, which limited the destructive tendencies, but did nothing to help ease Toby's actual anxiety. Erin even paid for a dog trainer to assess Toby and teach her how to provide stability and security that he so clearly needed.

As a rescue, no one could tell Erin what the root of his anxiety was. No one knew what his life was like before Erin adopted him. And as time went on, his anxiety got worse and worse. Erin could not even rearrange her furniture. If she did, Toby behaved as if he did not recognize the room, as if he had never been in that room before.

At one point, Toby's anxiety led him to begin hurting himself. He started self-mutilating, chewing at his feet and tail until they bled. He started trying to chew his way out of his crate whenever he was left alone, which led to several chipped or broken teeth that had to be removed by a veterinarian. At one point, he even chewed up a container of boot wax, which seemed harmless enough until Erin provided the list of ingredients (one of which was toxic) to the veterinarian. The boot wax incident led to a full week of hospitalization for Toby, which was both traumatic for Toby and expensive for Erin.

Finally, Erin decided to put Toby on a common anti-anxiety medication called Fluoxetine. Fluoxetine is the generic name for Prozac. Erin obtained a prescription for the medication from her veterinarian, but even after several months of constant use, and an increase in his dose, Erin saw little change with Toby's anxiety.

Then, a friend recommended that Erin reach out a local pet trainer with a background in holistic medicine. With nothing left to lose, Erin made an appointment, and she and Toby met with the trainer.

The trainer suggested that Erin gently wean Toby off of the Fluoxetine prescription, and begin using a variety of holistic therapies for anxiety. She recommended the popular "Thunder Shirt" for Toby to wear, as well as a few minor changes around their home to help Toby feel comfortable relaxed. But the most important recommendation she made was to start Toby on a CBD product specifically designed for dogs with anxiety.

That day, Erin went to her local dispensary and purchased a product called Therabis. Therabis was a CBD powder, designed to be sprinkled on a dog's food, for easy dosing. Erin began the CBD powder regimen immediately and crossed her fingers.

While Erin did not see results immediately, she did begin to see results after a few weeks of daily use. By the third month, Toby was a different dog, relaxed, comfortable, and shy but not terrified. Toby still had some very extreme reactions to stressful events in life, but his day-to-day quality of life was much improved. And as a result, Erin's quality of life was also improved.

At their next veterinary visit, Toby's doctor was astounded by his progress. Toby has now been on a strict CBD regimen for two years, and he is living a happy, healthy life with only mild-anxiety, instead of the tense, stressful life of constant-anxiety.

Chapter 3: Rick Simpson Oil

Rick Simpson was an engineer in Canada long before he was known for his cannabis-laced oil, now known as Rick Simpson Oil. In 1997, he was working in a hospital where he was treating asbestos with a very strong aerosol glue. Because the room was so poorly ventilated, Simpson inhaled a large amount of the toxic fumes and collapsed. The fumes had caused his nervous system to go into shock, and when he collapsed, he fell off his ladder and hit his head. The fall knocked him unconscious, and when he woke up, he found himself in the emergency room.

After the incident, Simpson started to hear a ringing in his ears and began experiencing dizzy spells. This went on for years, and no matter what medication he was prescribed, his symptoms never improved, in fact, they got worse.

Years later, Simpson happened to see a documentary that highlighted the benefits of cannabis and the many medicinal properties associated with it. He contacted his doctor to inquire about medical marijuana, but the doctor refused to prescribe it to him. As a result, Simpson chose to obtain marijuana on his own. Once he started to use it, he noticed a marked improvement in the ringing in his ears (known as tinnitus), as well as other symptoms.

Simpson continued to use marijuana to treat his tinnitus and dizzy spells, and in 2003, he noticed three new, odd-looking bumps appear on his arm. His doctor suspected the bumps may be cancerous, and a biopsy was performed. Simpson was diagnosed with Basal Cell Carcinoma, a form of skin cancer.

Simpson, in consideration for the way marijuana had helped him treat his tinnitus and dizzy spells, began doing some research. He found a study that reported THC used in mice led to the death of cancer cells in those mice. This study was published in the Journal of the National Cancer Institute. After reading this study, Simpson decided to start treating his Basal Cell Carcinoma with a topical cannabis treatment. To do this, he developed a concentrated cannabis oil.

Simpson would apply this oil to a bandage and would apply the bandage to his carcinoma for several days. After four days of use, the bandages were removed, and Simpson noted that the cancerous growth had disappeared.

Of course, Simpson's doctor refused to acknowledge that it was the cannabis oil treatments that successfully cured the carcinoma. At the time, cannabis use was still considered prohibitive, and very few doctors were willing to acknowledge or discuss the medicinal properties of cannabis, THC, and CBD.

Simpson, of course, was a true believer at this point. He began to do more and more research and even started cultivating and harvesting his own marijuana plants for use in his research. He developed a specialized strain of cannabis and began making a "cannabis concentrate" from that plant. This concentrate has become known as "Rick Simpson Oil" or "RSO."

As a result of his marijuana cultivating, marijuana use, and his decision to provide this concentrated oil to cancer patients (free of charge), he faced persecution from the Canadian authorities. He was arrested multiple times, his home was repeatedly raided, and his plants were continuously destroyed and/or confiscated by the Royal Canadian Mounted Police. Regardless of these setbacks,

Simpson knew his concentrated oil could be a literal live saver, so he insisted on continuing with his work.

While Rick Simpson Oil can be purchased at local dispensaries, it is also possible to make your own version of Rick Simpson Oil at home. Although we must warn you, the ingredients required to make Rick Simpson Oil at home may not be legal, depending on which state you live in.

The process of creating a concentrated cannabis oil is actually pretty simple, and it is not difficult to make. First, you should choose the marijuana strain that best suite you. True Rick Simpson Oil uses indica strains, but you may use indica or sativa, whichever you prefer.

The recipe we are about to share should produce a full sixty grams of the concentrated oil. This is enough for a ninety-day treatment plan. You can always make smaller batches, just do as you would if you were baking cookies. Cut the recipe in half, or thirds, or even more, whatever suits your needs. For reference, a single ounce of cannabis typically produces four grams of concentrated oil.

Ingredients:
- Isopropyl alcohol, 99%, Two gallons
- Dry indica cannabis, one pound
- A wooden spoon
- A syringe, with a catheter tip, 60mL size recommended
- A rice cooker
- A large bowl
- A cheesecloth
- A bucket, five gallons

1. First, put your dry cannabis into the bucket and pour the isopropyl alcohol on it until all of the dried plant material is covered.
2. Mix the combination well, crushing the plant as you stir. Stir the mixture for three to four minutes, allowing the cannabis to dissolve into the alcohol. You should note that nearly eighty percent of the cannabis will dissolve.
3. Using the cheesecloth, strain all of the isopropyl alcohol out of the cannabis material.
4. Move your cannabis material back to the bucket, and add more of the isopropyl alcohol to it again, stirring and crushing it as you did before.
5. Again, using your cheesecloth, strain the alcohol out of the mixture.
6. Take the strained solvent and pour it into your rice cooker. Do not fill your rice cooker more than three-quarter of the way full. Turn the rice cooker on.
7. Keep the rice cooker temperature between 200 and 250 degrees (Fahrenheit), as this is the necessary temperature for decarboxylation to occur. If you heat it above 300 degrees, the cannabinoids you want to extract will actually cook off or burn off, rendering your concentration oil useless. Using a slow cooker (like a Crockpot) will likely overheat your cannabis product.
8. The alcohol will evaporate as the rice cooker heats up. Slowly add your cannabis mix to the rice cooker, and make sure to keep the rice cooker in a well-ventilated area. Obviously, because isopropyl alcohol is flammable, avoid keeping your rice cooker near stovetops, open flames, cigarettes, or other forms of fire/sparks.
9. Once all of the alcohol has evaporated, you should be left with a thick oil. Using your 60mL catheter-tip syringe, draw the oil out of the pan and into the

syringe. This is the easiest and cleanest method, especially as you can dispense the oil straight from the syringe.

So, why should you use Rick Simpson Oil? While we strongly recommend that you seek the opinion of your doctor, there is a strong chance that your doctor will not be willing to discuss the oil with you, as many cannabis or CBD products exist in a grey area, legally.

The typical recommendation for Rick Simpson Oil is for a patient to consume 60 grams of the oil over a period of ninety days, following a scheduled pattern.

Days 1 through 7:
Use the oil three times a day, every day. Each dose should be no larger than a half grain of rice, and each dose should be taken eight hours apart.

Days 8 through 35:
Every four days, you should double your dose, until you are eventually taking one full gram of Rick Simpson oil each day. Most people do not reach this point until they have been using the Rick Simpson oil for a full five weeks.

Days 36 through 90:
Continue consuming one full gram of Rick Simpson oil each day until you have consumed a total of 60 grams. This will likely mean taking eight or nine drops (each the size of a rice grain) every eight hours.

Now, the reason it takes some people many weeks before they can consume a full gram of Rick Simpson oil in one day is simply because of the way it tastes. The oil is typically very bitter so you may want to mix it with a food like a yogurt to hide the bitter taste.

The side effects of Rick Simpson Oil are minimal, and most people only experience a bit of sleepiness. Most users report that the sleepiness goes away after four weeks of consistent use.

Once you complete the ninety-day course, it is important to keep Rick Simpson oil on hand. You will likely only need to use a gram or two of the oil each month to maintain your results.

But remember, it is not a cure-all. It has been found to be effective in treating many skin-related issues, and it can provide significant relief, but it will not cure your condition.

TESTIMONIAL

John was only thirty-two when he noticed a small mole on his forearm had begun to change shape and color. At the advice of his wife, he had the mole examined by a doctor, and it was quickly diagnosed as Melanoma.

John knew too much about cancer—chemotherapy and the harsh, life-altering medications often prescribed by doctors when treating cancerous conditions. John knew that those treatments would be hard on his body and immune system, and he had seen friends and family members go through it. He knew that they almost always felt worse after those treatments and that it was an incredibly difficult path.

John asked his doctor about alternative options for treatment and was met with a wealth of resistance. His doctor did not want him to pursue unconventional treatments. His doctor insisted that the only appropriate course of treatment was the conventional chemotherapy treatments.

Refusing to put himself through the veritable hell that he saw his friends and family members go through with cancer treatments, John pursued alternative treatments anyway. He changed his diet, began exercising, and started seeing a Naturopath. Eventually, his wife found an article online, citing the benefits of Rick Simpson Oil, and showed it to John. He was skeptical and likened the product to "snake oil" or a placebo. But as his wife put it, "What could it hurt to try it?"

They located a local dispensary, and while the dispensary did not carry the product on their shelves, they were more than willing to order the product for John. Within a few weeks, and for a price much lower than the cost of a chemotherapy treatment, John had a bottle of Rick Simpson Oil in his hand.

He followed the directions closely for the ninety-day course of treatment and took photographs of his mole along the way. Within four weeks, the mole appeared smaller in size. Within eight weeks, the mole's color began to fade. And on day seventy-five, the mole was no longer visible.

To be on the safe side, John completed the ninety-day course, even though his mole was no longer visible after day seventy-five. He returned to his doctor a mere five months after the diagnosis, and his doctor was amazed.

His doctor is now a true believer in the power of CBD Oil, and while he cannot legally recommend CBD oil to his patients, he does now encourage his patients to pursue alternative therapies, and he often implies that he has known patients to see success with the use of CBD oil.

And when it comes to Rick Simpson oil in particular, there are hundreds if not thousands of personal testimonies to be found online, all of which tout the cancer-reducing benefits of the concentrated CBD tar/oil treatment. Just take a quick look at the Rick Simpson Oil website, and we are sure you will agree with us that Rick Simpson Oil is worth trying.

Chapter 4: Cannabis Legalities & Products

As we mentioned earlier in the book, marijuana is nothing if not controversial. As a result, any product associated with marijuana is also controversial. We have already discussed which states allow medical or recreational marijuana, and where CBD sits among those regulations and legislation.

THC and CBD are the two primary compounds that can be extracted from marijuana. Other cannabinoids exist and can also be extracted, but they exist in such small amounts and are so rarely extracted for products, that they are not really a concern. In any event, there have been many studies that show CBD, in particular, have anti-inflammatory properties.

The types of CBD products available on the market are intended to reach a wide variety of consumers. You can find just about anything, from oils and tinctures to beauty products, to products meant for your canine companion. As we discussed before, every state handles CBD products differently. CBD products that do not contain any level of THC are completely legal in every state, but they may have restrictions placed on them related to who can sell them and where.

If you are interested in knowing which CBD products are recommended, here is a list of the various products that we found to have five-star reviews:

- CW Hemp's Everyday Advanced Hemp Oil
- Herb Essntls' Moisturizer
- Infinite CBD Vaporizer
- Cibaderm Shampoo
- Kiva's Ginger Dark Chocolate

- Sacred Biology Deodorant
- Pure Kana Premium CBD Drops
- Mary Medicinals Transdermal Patch
- Wildflower CBD+ Capsules
- CBD For Life Face & Body Wash
- Rick Simpson Oil
- Therabis "Calm & Quiet" Powder for Dogs
- Therabis "Up & Moving" Powder for Dogs
- Therabis "Stop The Itch" Powder for Dogs

Looking for a reputable manufacturer of CBD cannabinoid products? The following companies have been reviewed by independent source online and have fantastic reviews. To purchase a product from one of these manufacturers, simply contact your local dispensary and ask if they carry it or if they can order it for you:

- Zamnesia
- Zakah Life Essentials
- ViPova
- Vape Bright
- Trompetol
- TreatWell
- Treatibles
- Therapy Pure Essentials
- Therabis
- The Medics
- The Fay Farm
- Tasty Hemp
- SoS Pain Relief
- Smart Organics
- Sagely Natural
- Sadica
- Receptra Naturals
- PyoorCBD
- Purity Petibles
- Hygia Nutrients
- Holy Grail
- Holland Hemp Company
- Highland Pharms
- HempWorx
- Hemp Power
- Hemp Meds
- HempLucid
- Hemplogica
- Hempland
- Hemp Health Technologies
- Hemp Fusion
- Hemp Forte
- Green Roads
- Green Gorilla
- Green Garden Gold
- Gevitta
- Folium Biosciences

- Pure Spectrum
- Pure Ratios
- Pure CBD Vapors
- Pura Vida
- Prime My Body
- Populum
- PH Secrets
- Phivida
- PharmaHemp
- Palmetto Harmony
- Organabus
- Nulief
- NuLeaf Naturals
- Noontide Herbal Elixirs
- Nectar Leaf
- Nature's Way Botanicals
- NanoCraft
- Muscle Rx
- Miracle Smoke
- Michigan Hemp Company
- Medihemp
- Mary's Medicinals
- Mana Artisan Botanics
- LoveCBD
- Lidtke
- Koi CBD
- Kiva Confections
- Kannaway
- KanaVape
- Isodiol
- Irie CBD
- iPuff
- Entourage Hemp
- Endoca
- Elixinol
- Elite Botanicals
- Dose of Nature
- Dixie Botanicals
- Diamond CBD
- Delta Botanicals
- Crystal Pure CBD
- Cloud 9 Hemp
- Cibdol
- CibDex
- Cibaderm
- CBDfx
- CBD Fusion Water
- Casa Luna Chocolate
- CannazAll
- Canna-Pet
- Cannadiol
- Canna Companion
- CanChew Gum
- C.W. Botanicals
- Blue Moon Hemp
- Bluebird Botanicals
- Bio Hemp
- BioCBD
- Arisitol
- AON Mother Nature
- Amrita
- Amma Life
- American Shaman
- Alaska Cannabis Exchange
- Aceso
- 4 Corners Cannabis

- iHemp

Each of the aforementioned companies is considered a reputable source for your CBD products, and I can speak from personal experience when I tell you that many of these companies have their products featured at the local dispensaries where I live.

Did you know there are even beauty products that contain CBD? From makeup to moisturizers to shampoo, if you can think of a product, odds are that you can find that product with CBD infused in it.

Remember, when it comes to CBD products, you will face greater legislation and restrictions in the following states, as these states prohibit marijuana use:

Wyoming	*Nebraska*
Wisconsin	*Missouri*
Virginia	*Mississippi*
Utah	*Kentucky*
Texas	*Kansas*
Tennessee	*Iowa*
South Dakota	*Indiana*
South Carolina	*Idaho*
Oklahoma	*Georgia*
North Carolina	*Alabama*

In addition, you will face greater restrictions and limitations if you try to purchase CBD products online. Because marijuana is illegal on the Federal level, that makes the transportation of marijuana products from one state to another illegal, even if one or both states allow the medical or recreational use of marijuana. Transporting marijuana products across state lines is a federal crime that could lead to prison time and a substantial fine.

As we said before, CBD products are legal to use provided there is no THC cannabinoid in the same product. If you purchase a CBD product that does not provide a detailed ingredient label, or if the police officer involved does not believe what is written on the label of the confiscated product, you could be arrested and/or charged with possession of marijuana. Only after the product has been tested—and the test has proven that it does not contain THC—will the charges be dropped.

Because of this, you need to be incredibly careful about which CBD products you purchase and where you purchase them from. Many, many studies have shown that CBD is more effective when they are paired with THC, so many CBD products, therefore, include THC. Legally, if the product contains more than 0.3% THC, it is considered a marijuana product, and it is subject to marijuana legislation.

If the product contains less than 0.3% THC, make sure that the manufacturer has a good reputation and stronger consumer reviews. Many research studies have been focused on ingredient testing, and have found that the amounts of CBD and/or THC are substantially different than what is listed on the label.

So, why do you need to be so incredibly cautious? Because marijuana legislation is *strict*. The penalty for trafficking marijuana depends on how much you are caught with, and whether or not it is your first offense.

If you are caught with 1000 kg or more of marijuana plants or marijuana "mixtures," you could face ten years or more in a federal prison and up to a $10 million dollar fine for your first offense, or twenty years or more in a federal prison, and up to a $20 million dollar fine for a second offense. If they determine that death or bodily injury occurred as a result of your trafficking, you could face life in prison.

If you are caught with more than 100 kg or less than 999 kg, you could face five years or more in a federal prison for a first offense, or ten years or more in a federal prison and up to a $20 million dollar fine. Again, if they determine that death or bodily injury occurred, you could face life in prison.

If you are caught with 50 kg to 99 kg of marijuana, you could face no more than twenty years in federal prison and a $1 million fine for the first offense, or no more than thirty years in a federal prison, and a $2 million fine for a second offense. If death or bodily injury occurred as a result, you could face life imprisonment.

If you are caught with less than 50kg of marijuana, you could face no more than five years in a federal prison and a fine of $250,000 for a first offense, or no more than ten years in prison and a $500,000 fine for a second offense.

For reference, 50 kg is equal to approximately 110 pounds. In addition, hashish and other marijuana or cannabis products that are not pure or true THC are still considered illegal under federal law. You should be just as cautious about purchasing CBD products, or any other cannabinoid product (like CBC or CBG), as you are about purchasing THC products. It is better safe than sorry!

HOW TO OBTAIN A MEDICAL MARIJUANA CARD

Each state that allows medical marijuana use has slightly different regulations that outline which conditions qualify for medical marijuana use. To obtain a medical marijuana card, you first have to be diagnosed with one of the qualifying conditions by a licensed medical professional.

Now, it is important to remember that your doctor does not give your medical marijuana card, and he does not "prescribe" the card to you. He simply diagnoses your condition and provides you with documentation related to that diagnosis, so that you can submit that documentation to your state, along with your Medical Marijuana Card application.

The following illnesses or conditions qualify under most state regulations:

- seizures or epilepsy
- muscle spasm disorders
- Multiple Sclerosis
- HIV (Human Immunodeficiency Virus)
- Hepatitis C
- glaucoma
- Crohn's Disease
- chronic pain
- chronic nausea
- cancer
- cachexia
- Alzheimer's Disease
- ALS (Amyotrophic Lateral Sclerosis)
- AIDS (Acquired Immune Deficiency Virus)

We strongly encourage you to contact your state's Department of Health or do some research online, to determine if your state recognizes your condition as a qualifying condition for Medical Marijuana use.

STEP 1:

- You must establish a physician-patient relationship with a physician that is licensed to practice in your state. This doctor can be a traditional doctor (MD), a homeopathic doctor (MD/H or OD/H), an osteopathic doctor (DO), or a naturopathic doctor (ND or NMD).

STEP 2:

- Once that relationship has been established, you will need to ask your doctor to complete and sign a Medical Marijuana Certification form. Do not use any random form that you found online. Make sure the form you are using is specific to your state. Also, a simple, written recommendation will not be enough. It has to be the state-certified form.

STEP 3:

- The physician that signs the form does not need to be the same physician that diagnosed you with the qualifying illness, but they will need access to your previous medical records to review that diagnosis.

STEP 4:

- With your signed state certification form in hand, you can now begin collecting the documentation you will need to complete the rest of the paperwork. You will need to provide proof of your residency in your state. This can be done with your Driver's License, your Passport, or any other state- or federally-issued photo identification.
- You may also need to provide a current photograph of yourself. This photograph must be taken within

sixty days of your application and must be taken without hats, glasses, or anything else that might obscure the view of your full face. The safest bet is to have a new "passport" photo taken.

- If you participate in SNAP (Supplemental Nutrition Assistance Program, a program sponsored by the USDA), you may need to provide documentation of your SNAP eligibility and current benefits.

STEP 5:

- These documents then need to be scanned into a PDF format, so that you can upload them to your state's website and submit them with your Patient Attestation Form, as directed by your state's Department of Health.

STEP 6:

- You must now register with your state's Department of Health, and submit your documents and certified forms to the Department of Health. This is typically done online, although some states may require you to mail these documents into their office.

Now, how much does a Medical Marijuana Card cost? Each state has different regulations, which means that each state has different fees. On average, the application fee is around $150.00. If you participate in SNAP, you may only need to pay $75-$100 for the application fee.

In addition, there is typically a $200 fee for the "registry identification card." This means that you should expect to pay approximately $350 in state fees and approximately $100-200 in doctor's fees. You should budget $500 to $750 to obtain your Medical Marijuana card. In addition, be prepared for the cost of medical marijuana. Many products are expensive. Check with your local dispensaries about their prices, and perhaps consider traveling to a large city where there are many dispensaries, to get products at the best possible price.

If you are interested in opening a Marijuana dispensary of your own, the fees are even higher, $500 to register as a dispensary agent, $5000 for the dispensary registration certificate, $1000 to renew that certificate, $2500 if you need to move your dispensary to a new location, and other fees, as well.

These fees are obviously independent of the cost of your visits to your doctor's office. You will need to pay the appropriate fees to get established with your doctor, to have them sign the appropriate certification form, and then you may need to pay fees if you need to obtain a new license, a new photograph or other documentation.

Obtaining a medical marijuana card is not cheap, and there are a lot of hoops you will need to jump through to obtain it. Unfortunately, you cannot simply tell your doctor that you have anxiety and then walk out of that office with a Medical Marijuana card in your hand.

The process is expensive, time-consuming, and involved, and the approval of your application makes take weeks to happen.

The most important points to remember when you are considering purchasing marijuana are as follows:

1. *If you live in a state where all marijuana use is prohibited, DO NOT purchase marijuana in another state and then bring it home with you. This is*

considered "drug trafficking," and it is a federal crime.

2. *If you live in a state that only allows medical marijuana use, and you do not have a valid Medical Marijuana Card for your state, DO NOT purchase recreational marijuana in another state and then bring it home with you. Again, this is considered "drug trafficking," and it is a federal crime.*

3. *Medical Marijuana Cards are only valid in the state they were originally issued in. If your card was issued in Arizona, that does not make it valid in Montana.*

4. *Crossing state lines with marijuana in your possession is a major risk, even if you have the proper documentation or a valid medical marijuana card. There will always be a question as to the legality of what you are transporting, and if you are caught moving marijuana from one state to another, you could face federal charges.*

What about marijuana or cannabis use in Europe?

For many, many years, Prague has held an annual cannabis festival, called Cannafest. Over the last five years, visitors of Cannafest have noted an impressive increase in the number of hemp or CBD products available at Cannafest, from drops to tinctures to oils to capsule to balms and more. In addition, countries like the Czech Republic have seen CBD products flood their commercial markets and become readily available and easily accessible.

Jiri Novak is the CEO of a "Canna b2b," a cannabis marketing company. When speaking of Cannafest, he said that everyone seems to be into CBD products now and that they are now seeing producers from Germany, Slovenia,

Denmark, Poland, and Holland, including the expected Czechia.

CBD is completely legal throughout Europe, with the only exception being Slovakia. Much of the research that has been done on CBD has been done in Europe. As a result, there are a wealth of European farmers that are taking full advantage of the CBD market boom and new research. They are making more money than ever before now that they can cultivate products beyond the traditional hemp seeds and fiber.

Many of these European cannabis curators have tried to export their products to the United States, especially now that so many of those states have legalized some form of marijuana or cannabis use. However, because cannabis is still prohibited by the Federal government, the United States Food & Drug Agency has prohibited any and all unapproved cannabidiol products.

As it currently stands, CBD products are legally prohibited from including any other cannabinoid, whether it is THC, CBC or CBG. This is especially frustrating, as it takes a lot of work to extract CBD from cannabis so completely that no other cannabinoid exists within the product. This is especially frustrating for consumers, as it limits the available product, and nearly all marijuana research indicates that cannabinoids are most effective when paired with another cannabinoid. These frustrations often lead CBD users to begin using regular marijuana, often obtained illegally.

The Czech Republic recently approved the use of cannabis sativa extracts in food-grade products. The only requirement is that the product should contain less than 0.15ppm of the THC cannabinoid.

Boris Banas, a board member with European Industrial Hemp Association (or EIHA), recently lectured about Europe's CBD laws. He stated that CBD products are often marketed within the food industry space, never mind that the label and declarations required by law do not exist within the food industry space. This makes CBD products incredibly difficult to regulate and control. CBD marketing is not helpful, either, as many CBD companies will deliberately label CBD products so that their product name is suspiciously close to the name of other cannabis products, often which carry high contents of THC. This is incredibly misleading and inappropriate, but without regulation, may never go away.

Chapter 5: The Dark Side of Cannabis

When marijuana was first legalized in Colorado, a rash of reports hit the news media that suggested marijuana use was contributing to higher rates of automobile accidents, emergency room visits, and drug overdoses throughout the state. This was the central argument used in other states whenever marijuana legislation was proposed.

In 2013, the American Psychiatric Association published an edition of the *Diagnostic and Statistical Manual of Mental Disorders* that listed three different cannabis-related issues that they were now considering as "mental disorders." These three issues were: cannabis intoxication, cannabis withdrawal, and cannabis-use disorder.

An associate professor of behavioral sciences and psychiatry at John Hopkins University School of Medicine, Ryan Vandrey, Ph.D., completed a study on the harmful use of cannabis, and the labeling and quality control issues that aid in such harmful use. Dr. Vandrey analyzed seventy-five samples and found that seventeen of those samples had significantly higher levels of THC than was listed (in some cases, more than ten percent more than was listed). Forty-five of the samples listed had significantly less THC than was listed.

In fact, one product analyzed was labeled to contain 1000 milligrams when it actually contained 1236 milligrams. Dr. Vandrey used these findings to encourage the community to adopt standardizations for the labeling and testing of marijuana or cannabis products.

The other concern noted by the American Psychiatric Association was the propensity that marijuana dispensaries have for adulterating or doctoring their products to boost sales. Some dispensaries have been found to mix glass crystals with their cannabis because a subtle "sparkle effect" can indicate a higher THC concentration than is truly there.

Once marijuana or cannabis becomes more mainstream and more legally acceptable throughout the United States, we suspect we will not only discover new uses for marijuana and cannabis products, but these products will certainly be more appropriately regulated in the future.

With proper regulations in place, there should be less fraudulent activity, which should cut down on the amount of accidental "overdoses," as well as the improving the quality of the products available on the market.

Marcel Bonn-Miller, the laboratory director at the Department of Veterans Affairs Substance & Anxiety Intervention Laboratory, has said that cannabis is a drug that is abused, and that science can demonstrate that abuse, as cannabis withdrawal has many of the same signs or symptoms as other drug withdrawals. He goes on to say that, for the most part, the symptoms of cannabis addiction or overuse are primarily behavioral. Bonn-Miller says that studies have found that as you are withdrawing from marijuana, you are likely to experience a decreased appetite or difficulty sleeping. These symptoms are most common during the first week of withdrawal but subside within a one month of withdrawal. Bonn-Miller went on to say that, since 2009, he has seen a marked increase in the inappropriate use of marijuana in Post-Traumatic Stress Disorder patients.

As we mentioned before, the most important point you can take away from reading this book is simply this: there has never been a proven or documented case of "cannabis overdose." The majority of the arguments that speak against marijuana use are concerned with addiction and overdose, but neither condition is a true factor in marijuana or cannabis use. Furthermore, CBD is non-intoxicating. They do *not* get you high, and again, there has never been a documented case of a CBD overdose or toxicity.

Granted, there are certainly going to be a few people that are allergic to marijuana, and it could cause an anaphylactic reaction in those people. But the odds of a marijuana allergy or cannabis allergy are very, very small. You are far more likely to be allergic to peanuts, strawberries or shellfish, or to have generalized environmental allergies.

Remember, the mutations of the endocannabinoid system are different in every person. Some people are more sensitive or receptive to cannabinoids than others, and some are less sensitive and receptive than others. This means that you may face a lot of trial and error when it comes to finding a CBD product that works for you—and a dose that works for you. You may also find that you need to increase your dose over time, as your body becomes more and more accustomed to the product, or you may need to change product formulations entirely.

TESTIMONIAL

Deborah is a grandmother of five. Her oldest grandchild, James, is a veteran of the Iraq war. He served three consecutive tours in the Middle East, and when he returned home, he was quickly diagnosed with Post-Traumatic Stress Disorder, anxiety, and depression. As a result of his illnesses, he found himself living in Deborah's home.

Deborah had been a lifelong advocate of the War Against Drugs. She had no tolerance for drug use of any kind, including alcohol, and when James moved into her home, she insisted that he maintain a clean and sober life. James agreed and began seeing a Psychiatrist regularly.

James' psychiatrist prescribed a number of medications to James, including an antidepressant, an anti-anxiety, and a medication to help him sleep. Even after months of therapy and consistent use of the medications he had been prescribed, James saw little relief.

Watching her grandson deteriorate was heartbreaking for Deborah. He began to lose weight and became more and more distant. His Post-Traumatic Stress Disorder seemed to get worse. The only way he could sleep was if he took the sleeping pills he had been prescribed, but those always led to night terrors.

James' quality of life was non-existent. He could not keep a job, he could not maintain a relationship, and his physical health was deteriorating just as quickly as his mental health.

Deborah finally decided to take matters into her own hands and started researching James' conditions and the various treatments. She saw that CBD use was something many people found success with, but she could not bring herself to allow him to use a marijuana product in her home.

It was not until James tried to take his own life that Deborah decided CBD would be a better alternative than his death. James spoke with his psychiatrist, who recommended trying CBD without THC first, but told

James he would be happy to put him in touch with a doctor that could help him obtain a Medical Marijuana card, if necessary.

James began using a CBD tincture right away. At the recommendation of his psychiatrist, he chose a tincture that was specifically formulated for anxiety and other mental illnesses. His results were not immediate, while the CBD did leave him feeling less "on edge," it took several weeks of consistent use before he started to see true results.

In a few short months, James was more relaxed, he was sleeping better, and he was learning to enjoy his life again. He was able to stop using sleeping pills all together, and he was able to find a good job. Within a year, James was able to wean himself off each of the prescription medications his Psychiatrist had prescribed, and all because of CBD oil!

Watching James heal and find a path to a healthier, more fulfilling life was all Deborah needed to forever change her mind about CBD Oil and the effects of marijuana. While recreational use of marijuana still makes Deborah uneasy, she is an outspoken and active advocate for using CBD to assist in improving mental health and helping heal the mind after traumatic experiences.

Conclusion: Review

Now, remember, CBD with THC is only legal in states that have legalized marijuana use, medically or recreationally. CBD without any THC is legal in all fifty states, but there may some restrictions within your state.

As we discussed previously, the legalities surrounding marijuana and CBD products are complicated. CBD products must contain less than 0.3% of the THC cannabinoid to be considered a legal, non-intoxicating product. In addition, states that prohibit the use of recreational marijuana have the right to confiscate your CBD product for testing to make sure the THC level listed is accurate. If it is not, and the product contains more than 0.3% THC levels, you could face federal charges related to the possession of marijuana, or even drug trafficking (which takes place any time you transport a drug across state lines).

If you live in a state that allows the use of recreational marijuana, you do not need to worry about whether or not your CBD products are legal, as long as you are purchasing them in the same state you live in.

If you live in a state that only allows the use of medical marijuana, you may want to obtain a Medical Marijuana Card, simply to protect yourself from a legal standpoint, should a CBD product in your possession be found to contain more than 0.3% of the THC cannabinoid. And again, you will want to make sure that the CBD products you purchase are purchased within the state you live in or have a Medical Marijuana card in.

Finally, if you live in a state that prohibits any and all marijuana use, you need to be very, very careful. You need to make sure that the CBD products you are purchasing are coming from a reputable manufacturer, and that you are purchasing these products within the same state you live in. You should not trust the CBD products you can find online, as they are almost certainly being shipped from outside your state.

These rules and regulations are sure to change as time goes on and more and more states legalize the use of marijuana, whether for recreational or medicinal purposes. If you intend to use CBD products long-term, we strongly recommend that you make a point to keep yourself educated on the changes to marijuana legislation. This legislation could change at any time, with little or no warning.

As it stands now, medical marijuana is legal in Washington D.C., Vermont, Washington, Hawaii, Rhode Island, Florida, Pennsylvania, Delaware, Oregon, Connecticut, Illinois, Colorado, Ohio, California, North Dakota, Arkansas, New York, Arizona, New Mexico, Alaska, New Jersey, Nevada, New Hampshire, Montana, Michigan, Minnesota, Massachusetts, Maine and Maryland. Meanwhile, West Virginia will allow the medical use of cannabis-infused products (like tinctures and oils), but not straight cannabis (like the dry herb). And Louisiana will allow the medical use of cannabis in any form except those forms that can be smoked.

Recreational marijuana use is legal in Washington D.C., Maine, Vermont, Colorado, Oregon, California, Nevada, Alaska, and Massachusetts. The only restrictions on recreational marijuana in these states are related to how much marijuana product you can carry and how many plants (if any) you are allowed to grow for personal use.

Marijuana is strictly prohibited in Wyoming, Kansas, Wisconsin, Iowa, Virginia, Indiana, Utah, Idaho, Texas, Georgia, Tennessee, Alabama, South Dakota, Oklahoma, South Carolina, North Carolina, Missouri, Nebraska, Mississippi, and Kentucky. Although, both Alabama and Mississippi will allow marijuana to be prescribed to medical patients diagnosed with severe epilepsy, a diagnosis that is very difficult to obtain.

These restrictions are important because, on a federal level, marijuana is still very illegal. As we have explained, CBD without THC is legal. But it can be difficult to obtain proof that the product is free of THC. Because of this technicality, you should be extremely cautious when you purchase your CBD products. Your safest option is to either move to a state that allows the recreational use of cannabis products or to obtain a Medical Marijuana card within the state of your residence. Obviously, these may not be options for everyone, but we have to advise it. We would hate for you to purchase a simple CBD product from a shady manufacturer and then face legal trouble for it.

CBD products have actually been used by humans in various cultures for approximately 10,000 years, even Queen Victoria used a CBD product to alleviate the pain and inflammation associated with her menstrual cycle, as well as for migraines. From "hemp fiber" used for weaving, to "hemp paper" used for map-making, to the more traditional CBD or Marijuana products you are used to hearing about, the marijuana plant has been used by humans for nearly a hundred centuries. These products are not new. And while we are only now discovering scientific evidence related to the many medicinal uses of CBD and the other cannabinoids, these medicinal uses have been suspected for as long as hemp or marijuana or cannabis has been used. These ideas are not new, though many of them have only recently been proven.

Marijuana or cannabis was not officially labeled as a dangerous drug until the Controlled Substances Act was passed in 1970. In fact, marijuana has only been officially illegal for forty-eight years! That means it was perfectly legal—although possibly frowned upon—when your grandparents were growing up!

Obviously, we have made greater strides when it comes to legalizing marijuana and hemp (or cannabis), but there is still a long, legal road ahead. Someday, we are sure, marijuana will be legal for both medical and recreational use, and there will be no question, anywhere, about the legality of hemp or cannabis products. Our greatest stride in the effort to protect cannabis products and distinguish them from marijuana or THC products was the Agricultural Act of 2014. This act, signed into law by President Barack Obama, now allows universities and research facilities to study and manufacture "industrial hemp."

Without this piece of legislation, CBD Oil would be even more controversial than it already is. As it stands, this legislation dictates that because the plant itself is legal (when the THC level is less than 0.3%), then any product made from that plant is also legal (as long as it has less than 0.3% THC).

In addition to these legalities, it is important to remember that CBD, and other cannabinoids like CBC and CBG, are non-intoxicating. THC is the only intoxicating cannabinoid we are aware of. Products that are free of THC will not cause intoxication or any sort of "high." Furthermore, in all of history, there has never been a record or confirmed death that resulted from marijuana or cannabis use. While you may experience some unpleasant side effects from using too much, it will not kill you.

As we discussed earlier, the sought-after side effects of CBD use include: anxiety relief, nausea relief, pain relief, reduced intraocular pressure or glaucoma, a slower rate of cancer growth, improved mood, lessened depression, and an overall peaceful feeling.

Some of the "negative" side effects of CBD cannabinoid use include lethargy, red eyes, irritated eyes, increased thirst or appetite, rapid heart rate, absentmindedness, dry mouth, dry eyes, coughing or bronchial irritation. In extreme cases, typically as a result of overuse or increased sensitivity, some side effects include paranoia or panic attacks.

These "negative" side effects are exceedingly rare and can often be avoided by simply using less of the CBD product in question. Everyone responds differently to CBD, so remember to start slowly. If you are using CBD products to assist with conditions like anxiety or insomnia, you may find that you develop a dependency on the product. This is not uncommon, and it does not necessarily mean that you are "addicted" to it. It simply means that you depend on that product to get to sleep at night, or to manage your anxiety. This is not any more dangerous than if a doctor prescribed to you an anti-anxiety medication or a sleeping pill and you became dependent on one of those medications (as most do).

The most important thing we can note here is CBD use has never been proven to cause death. There has been a reported or documented case of CBD toxicity or CBD-related death. Dependency will always be a concern, but it is up to you to determine whether or not you feel it is safer to depend on a CBD product or a medication prescribed by your doctor, which likely comes with a long list of serious side effects and medical warnings.

For those that are interested primarily in using CBD to treat cancer, we strongly recommend Rick Simpson Oil. Rick Simpson created this oil to treat his own Basal Cell Carcinoma, and his results were nothing short of impressive. His oil is now used by thousands of people to treat a variety of skin conditions, from cancer to acne to eczema and more. Rick Simpson Oil can be purchased at marijuana dispensaries, and there is a wealth of information, and plenty of testimonials, to be found on Rick Simpson's website.

And finally, if you are interested in using CBD products that contain THC, you may need to obtain a Medical Marijuana Card (unless you live in a state that has legalized recreational marijuana use). To obtain a Medical Marijuana card, you first need to be diagnosed with one of the qualifying illnesses or diseases, as defined by your state, and then you must find a doctor that is willing to complete and sign the state certified form. You cannot simply walk into a doctor's office and walk out with a prescription.

Obtaining a medical marijuana card is not easy, there is a lot of paperwork, and it may take weeks for the paperwork to be processed. It can also be very expensive. You may want to try using CBD-only products first. We think you will be surprised by how well they work on their own!

Cannabis research is in its infancy, we are sure to discover so much more about the plant over the next decade, from greater medical benefits to better product formulations, and more. As it is, CBD has been proven to help treat a myriad of illnesses or diseases, from anxiety to depression to post-traumatic stress disorder, from cancer to glaucoma to cachexia. It has even been shown to improve Alzheimer's and ALS. CBD may not be a cure-all, but there are thousands of people and hundreds of studies that all agree it was a beneficial treatment for their medical condition.

The first scientific studies to suggest that CBD could assist in relieving pain, nausea and anxiety were published in the 1980s, although they received little attention or acknowledgment until the 1990s. In 1998, we saw the first true breakthroughs in CBD research and manufacturing when G.W. Pharmaceuticals, a British company, started cultivating cannabis specifically for use in medical trials.

The research and cultivation performed by G.W. Pharmaceuticals led to other scientific studies performed by several collectives, including the International Cannabinoid Research Society, the International Association for Cannabinoid medicine, and the Society of Cannabis Clinicians. Many of these studies involved the study of how cannabinoids affected animals when used to treat anxiety and epilepsy.

By early 2009, a laboratory in California was able to successfully cultivate and grow strains of cannabis that held higher levels of CBD than THC, something that had previously been difficult to achieve.

CBD and their medicinal properties got even more attention in 2010 when a young family from Montana began using CBD oil to treat their toddler son's brain cancer. After intensive medical therapy, including over thirty rounds of radiation, the Hyde family began using CBD oil to treat the Stage 4 cancer because they had run out of other options. The brain tumor shrunk, and while there is no definitive proof that the CBD oil causes the tumor to shrink, no other changes were made that could indicate cause or effect. The CBD oil did not cure the young boy's cancer, but it did give his family an extra two years to spend with him before he eventually died as a result of his cancer.

The success of CBD oil was in headlines again in 2013, when a family began using CBD oil to treat their three-year-old's severe epilepsy. This little girl was experiencing approximately three hundred grand mal seizures every week, and the family had treated her condition with everything their doctors' recommended, from painful procedures to prescription medications. Nothing seemed to alleviate the seizures or the girl's suffering. After watching a documentary about medical marijuana, her parents decided to try CBD oil, and they were stunned to find that with using CBD oil, they were able to reduce their daughter's seizures by ninety-five percent. Instead of experiencing an average of three hundred seizures per week, the girl was only experiencing an average of fifteen seizures per week.

While there is not yet a wealth of scientific evidence to back up our claims about CBD and their various medicinal properties, there are thousands of personal testimonies and thousands of years of use and experience to back up our claims. CBD use produces so few side effects and negative reactions that is definitely worth trying if you suffer from pain, anxiety, insomnia, autoimmune conditions, cancer, or any of the other life-altering conditions mentioned in this book.

CBD Oil has had a positive effect on our lives, as well as the lives of many of our friends and family members. It has been used in one form or another for thousands of years, and we are finally conducting research to help prove that cannabis, marijuana, hemp, CBD, THC, CBC, CBG—all of these different varieties of the cannabis plant—can have life-altering and life-improving benefits for each and every one of us.

You have now reached the end of ***CBD & Cannabis Oil: The Essential Guide***. We sincerely hope that this book answered all of your questions about cannabis, THC, CBD, and more. If you found this book informative and helpful, we encourage you to leave us an honest review on Amazon. Thank you again for downloading this book!

Furthermore, please be advised that while we fully support the use of cannabis products (especially those with high concentrations of CBD) and that we are hopeful for a bright future in the cannabis industry, we obviously cannot guarantee that you will see the results you are hoping for. Everyone responds to cannabis, THC, CBD, CBC, CBG, and other hemp or cannabis products, differently. What worked for one person may not work for you, and it may require several rounds of "trial and error" before you find what works for you. But we strongly encourage you to try it! Cannabis treatments can be life-altering!

We sincerely hope that this book has helped you understand more about cannabis and the industry surrounding it. Many people have questions about cannabis, and many people do not understand that cannabis is not always intoxicating, or that intoxicating cannabinoids can be removed from the cannabis product, but they can! This makes a world of difference, especially when discussing the legalities. Marijuana, cannabis, hemp, whatever you may call it, could change the world! We hope you agree, and that you will join the fight to legalize cannabis products so that the world can be a happier, healthier place for everyone. After all, how can a plant that has existed as long as the Earth has existed—and that has been used by various cultures throughout the world since the very beginning of time—how can that product truly be unhealthy?

www.ingramcontent.com/pod-product-compliance
Lightning Source LLC
Chambersburg PA
CBHW070039260726
48658CB00002B/670